Not Just a Patient

How to Have a Life
When You Have
a Life-Threatening
Illness

by Ellen Fein

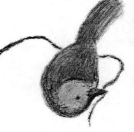

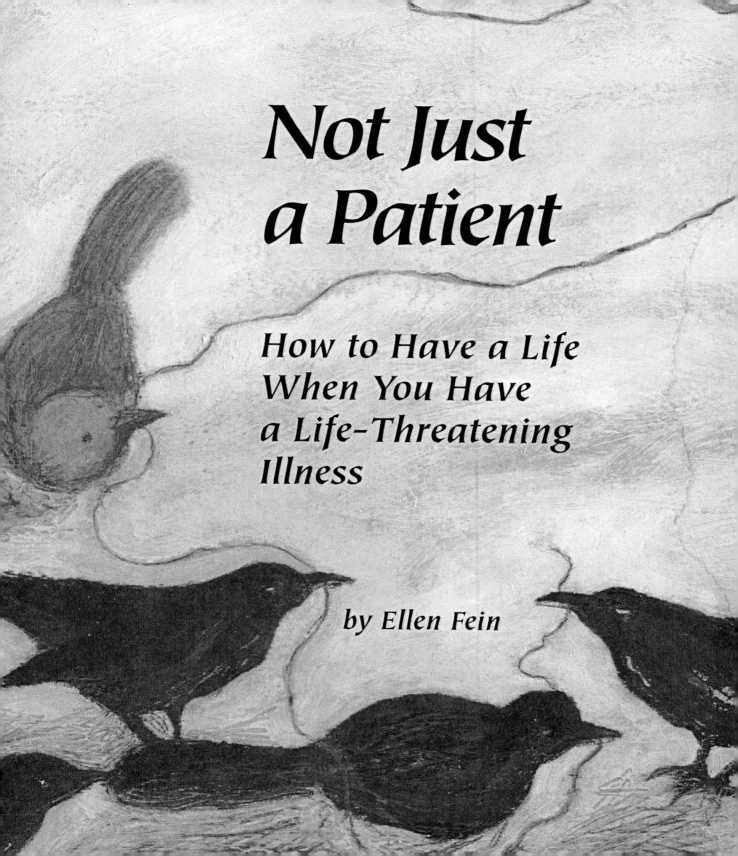

Not Just a Patient

How to Have a Life When You Have a Life-Threatening Illness

by Ellen Fein

Printed in Victoria, Canada

Editing by Rebecca Davison, Montpelier, Vermont
Design by Maureen O'Connor Burgess, Montpelier, Vermont
Photograph of author by Andrew Kline/afterimage photo, Montpelier, Vermont
Cover drawing by Carol MacDonald, Colchester, Vermont
Carol MacDonald is a professional artist and teacher who, along with exhibiting her work widely throughout the United States, conducts art and healing workshops. These workshops offer another way for people who are struggling with illness and grief to express themselves as they go through the healing process. The cover art portrays a magical moment when the birds realize they can pick up the string together. The image calls us to figure out new ways to nurture and support one another.

National Library of Canada Cataloguing in Publication Data

Fein, Ellen
Not just a patient : how to have a life when you have a life-threatening illness / Ellen Fein.
ISBN 1-55395-860-8

1. Sick--Psychology. 2. Adjustment (Psychology) 3. Self-care, Health. I. Title.
    R726.8.F43 2003   616'.001'9   C2003-901310-3

TRAFFORD

This book was published *on-demand* in cooperation with Trafford Publishing.
On-demand publishing is a unique process and service of making a book available for retail sale to the public taking advantage of on-demand manufacturing and Internet marketing. **On-demand publishing** includes promotions, retail sales, manufacturing, order fulfilment, accounting and collecting royalties on behalf of the author.

Suite 6E, 2333 Government St., Victoria, B.C. V8T 4P4, CANADA

Phone	250-383-6864	Toll-free	1-888-232-4444 (Canada & US)
Fax	250-383-6804	E-mail	sales@trafford.com
Web site	www.trafford.com	TRAFFORD PUBLISHING IS A DIVISION OF TRAFFORD HOLDINGS LTD.	
Trafford Catalogue #03-0223	www.trafford.com/robots/03-0223.html		

10   9   8   7   6   5   4   3   2

Dedication

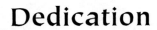

With deep love
and appreciation
to Michael Goldfinger
whose journey with cancer
and passage into death
taught so very much.

PREFACE

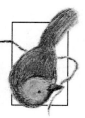

The idea for this book began in 1997 during the eight months my husband, Michael Goldfinger, lived with bone marrow cancer. For five of those months, he was actively engaged in treatment (including a bone marrow transplant), and for three months, he received hospice care. During that time we were lucky to discover many things that made our life surprisingly more comfortable and normal. Michael and I often passed on specific suggestions or fielded requests for information about what we had learned to other patients and families living with a life-threatening illness. Repeatedly, friends and acquaintances remarked that it was too bad there was no place to easily locate these kinds of tips for living. So, I had intended to write about this at some point, but as I went through my own grieving process and assumed my life as a single parent, I never got to it.

In December of 2000, just three years after Michael died, I was diagnosed with acute leukemia (AML), also a form of bone marrow cancer. I was hospitalized for over a month for treatment. Although I eventually was able to achieve a remission, my bone marrow failed to recover so I was unable to complete my treatment, which was essential if I was to sustain a remission. By late summer of 2001, it became clear that the only viable option for treatment was for me to have a stem cell transplant. In the fall, I moved with my teenage daughter and my partner to Seattle for four and a half months to undergo the transplant.

Shortly after my chemotherapy treatment, I decided to write this guide. I have drawn on all of my experience as both a caregiver and a patient and the experiences of many of the patients I have met along the way. The emphasis throughout the guide is on quality of life when undergoing medical treatment -- the things you can do to make your life have meaning beyond patienthood. These are things medical providers typically don't think about. This is not the definitive work. Even as we complete the final editing, I keep learning new tips that would be great to add.

Although I regularly use complementary/alternative health services, this guide is NOT focused on finding or using those. The focus is on life as a patient undergoing conventional medical treatment. I have, however, incorporated suggestions for how to integrate complementary practices in your life as a patient.

I use the word "healing" throughout this guide in the sense of well-being or wholeness. The meaning is not confined to the state of one's physical well being or by the stage of one's disease. Rather, it reflects the concept that health is based on the ability to incorporate the emotional, mental, spiritual, and social, as well the physical, aspects of one's life.

I firmly believe there are lots of actions -- some small and some not so small -- that you can take to make life work for you. This applies whether you are undergoing chemotherapy, radiation, or surgery; looking at an extended hospital stay or having outpatient care. I have written this in hopes it will make the lives of others easier.

Table of Contents

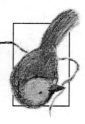

INTRODUCTION

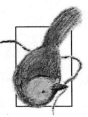

The Things You Need to Know That No One Tells You About Living

When you are diagnosed with a life-threatening illness, it is all too easy to find yourself transformed into a "PATIENT." You seem to lose your identity.

My experience during my husband's bone marrow cancer, and now my own, convinced me that you CAN have a life. You can retain much of the identity you had before you were ill, and as important, you can exercise a surprising amount of influence over and control of your treatment and treatment environment.

This guide is based on the following assumptions:

- Each person must pursue healing in a way that fits with who he or she is. What is the right choice for one patient may not be the right choice for someone else.

- In the end, only the patient is in a position to make treatment choices. Opinions from those who care and data from providers may be useful, but the patient has to choose treatment.

- Health care providers tend to focus on symptoms, blood counts, tumor markers, etc. Their attention is, most often, medical intervention and NOT quality of life.

- The patient can do a great deal to maintain that quality of life throughout treatment and during the course of a life threatening illness.
- The suggestions in this guide are just that -- suggestions. Some may seem helpful to the reader and others may seem way off base. I invite you to use what you want and disregard the rest.

TAKING CARE OF YOURSELF

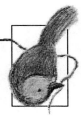

While you may turn over some important aspects of your health care to your doctor or health care provider, only you can attend to some key aspects of your health. When you do not feel well, it is easy to get overwhelmed by your own sense of illness. You can lessen this feeling and increase your sense of well-being. There are things that you can do that will help you face whatever is in front of you.

The Emotional Side

You will undoubtedly experience a wide range of feelings when you are diagnosed and as you live with your illness. Extreme feelings are a normal response. Sometimes, it can seem as if you are on an emotional roller coaster. Finding some balance can be very challenging. Living with lots of intense emotions may very well be part of your life now.

If you have coping strategies that normally work for you, use those (for example, exercise or prayer). You may also need some new strategies. When my husband was ill, I felt that the practice of yoga saved my sanity. And during my own illness, I have started meditating. Both of these have helped me gain some internal sense of balance even as external circumstances have been very unpredictable and/or trying.

For many, counseling really helps. If you want to find a resource, look for someone who is licensed in your state and who is experienced in working with individuals with serious health problems.

And, you should expect those around you will have their own emotions to deal with. Each of them will also need to find a way to live with their own feelings and get emotional support. Even though it is tempting to provide that support yourself, this is generally not realistic.

Cautions About Your "Attitude"

You will likely be bombarded with messages about how you should feel and what your attitude should be. These can be extremely detrimental. Take note of them, but do not lose track of your own sense of what is right and how you feel.

There will be those who tell you that you caused your own illness. There are any number of "experts" who promote the idea that emotions and stress cause illness. Lots of people experience as much stress or more than you, and they do not end up with a life-threatening illness.

Beware of the notion that having a positive attitude will cure your illness. No doubt there is a connection between our minds and our bodies, but if positive attitude were all it took to recover from a life-threatening illness, many fewer people would actually die.

Beware of the concept of the "exceptional patient" -- these are supposedly patients who get well because they take charge of their treatment and have a positive attitude. Each of us does the best we can. And for some of us, that seems simply ordinary. And sometimes we are down right unhappy or even nasty. This does not mean we cannot heal.

The Physical Side

Sleep, food, and exercise are important parts of staying healthy. When you have a life-threatening illness, it can be particularly hard to maintain these ingredients of health, but they are important for your healing. Although it is not my intent to offer specific advice, be sure to make room in your life with an illness to get adequate sleep, to maximize your nutritional intake, and to exercise as much as you are able.

A Word About Fear

It is all too easy to become afraid. Afraid of the effects of treatment. Afraid of anticipated pain. Afraid of death. Afraid about what might happen to those who will be left behind if you die. Most of us deal with our fear by trying not to think about it or trying to talk ourselves into being positive. It takes a lot of energy to do this, and the knot of fear never really goes away. For me, a clue that I am feeling afraid is a particular type of tightness in my stomach.

Consider trying something different. Let yourself contemplate the things you are afraid of. Let them see the light of your own awareness, and you may be surprised to see them change, and the fear may well lessen

MEDICAL INFORMATION

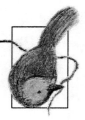

Deciding How Much You Want to Know

For some of us, getting information helps us cope. For others, it can be over-whelming or too discouraging. What is going to be most helpful for you? Each of us has to figure that out for ourself. Not an easy task when everything is so unknown and unpredictable. As early into the process as you can, think about how much and what type of information you want.

Do you want to know the survival odds? If the odds are not in your favor, how do you think it might affect you? Could it make you feel doomed? Will you be able to see that the numbers, while useful, are only just that? Numbers. If you want to get a great perspective on statistics and odds, check out this article by Stephen Jay Gould, *"The Median Isn't the Message"* at *http://cancerguide.org/median_not_msg.html*.

Are you going to want to have choices or would you prefer a single recommen-dation from your doctor? Some individuals feel empowered by gathering a lot of infor-mation and making a selection while others can be completely overwhelmed by need-ing to make decisions.

Preparing to See Your Health Care Provider

Before you go to see your health care provider, spend time preparing. Anticipate the range of subjects about which you want information. After you have determined what you want to know, organize and write down your questions. Given the anxiety that one has about seeing a health care provider under these circumstances, it is easy to forget to ask something. Taking a list of questions with you will help to minimize that possibility.

Below are some of the kinds of information you may want to get.

The Diagnosis. Are there questions about it? Do you fully understand what it means? If not, what else do you need to know? What might the progression of this illness look like? Keep in mind that sometimes a diagnosis represents a cluster of similar types of illnesses, particularly with some types of cancers. So, often, it is important to find out about your specific subtype.

Treatment. Are there any choices? What type of medicine and procedures are likely? Is there a standard treatment? If not, how will a treatment plan be developed? Where will the treatment occur? Is there a preferred location or provider? Will these factors make a difference to the outcome? How long will the treatment probably take? What are the likely side effects? What can be done for those? What kind of support will you need? Are there any experimental treatments available? Are there any government sponsored clinical trials that are testing new drugs or treatment strategies? If so, are you eligible to participate?

Support Services. What types of non-medical care might you need? Are there patient support groups or counseling services available? Could you talk to someone else with the same diagnosis?

Symptom Management. What kind of pain might you expect? How do you know when the pain is enough to warrant intervention? Will you have other physical discomfort? Side effects? How can those be managed?

Prognosis. How long do people with this diagnosis usually live? Do some people get a remission?[1] Do some people get cured?[2] In the medical world, cure may mean you really are disease free for the rest of your life or it may mean you are disease free for 3 or 5 years. If your provider uses the term "cure," ask that it be defined for you. If the provider has talked about remission, what does that mean? How long might you expect to be in remission? If the provider is recommending treatment that will not lead to a remission, will it extend your life? If so, by how much? Or might it lessen your pain or discomfort?

Using an Advocate

If you can, find someone who can be your advocate in this process. Ideally, this would be someone who will be able to think clearly and objectively. Possibly a spouse, another family member, or a friend could be the right person to help you.

The advocate's job is threefold:

1. To help you prepare for your appointments by thinking through what you want to know and to actually assist in creating a list of questions.

2. To assist at the appointment by making sure you get all of your questions asked, by actually recording the answers to the questions, and by asking for clarification if any of the answers are unclear.

3. And lastly, to help you process what you learn.

---

1. A remission is generally considered to be any period of time in which there is an absence of evidence of disease.

2. A cure is generally considered to mean a life that will remain disease free.

Getting and Remembering Information/Answers

When you get to your appointment, make sure that you ask all of the questions on your list and write down the answers. Take your time and go carefully down the list you prepared. Ask questions if you do not understand the answer. It is really easy to leave the appointment not having been able to remember or digest what has been said. This is where an advocate is very helpful.

You might also consider taking along a tape recorder. Whether or not someone goes with you, a tape recorder will help you remember what was said during the appointment. It is pretty difficult to take in and digest medical information and, at the same time, write down the answers to your questions.

You need not worry about how the provider will react to either the advocate or the tape recorder. It has been my experience that most providers want to make sure you understand as much as possible and will support you to make that happen.

Getting More Than One Opinion

It is always appropriate to get a second opinion when you are dealing with a life-threatening illness. You can ask your doctor for a recommendation and referral. Ideally that second opinion should be from someone who deals extensively with your illness. You want someone who has seen and treated many patients with your diagnosis.

There are many other avenues to healing besides traditional, Western medicine. You may also want to consider another opinion from a complementary or alternative medicine (often referred to as CAM) provider. Complementary providers are those that offer services that can be used in conjunction with traditional medicine and alternative providers are used instead of traditional medicine.

It is quite likely that you will have to do your own CAM research to identify what type of treatment might be worth considering. Unfortunately there is not the same kind of research base for complementary/alternative health care as there is for traditional Western medicine. Nonetheless, many people have found that these non-traditional services have been a key component in their own healing.

It is not my intent to evaluate or present detailed information on complementary and alternative medicine, but two good references can be found in *Choices in Healing: Integrating the Best of Conventional and Complementary Approaches to Cancer* by Michael Lerner and *Comprehensive Cancer Care* by Jim Gordon. Another resource is the National Institute for Health's complementary medicine web site at *http://nccam.nih.gov/*. CAM can include the following: exercises that calm your mind and emotions (yoga, meditation, relaxation, imagery); body and energy work (Therapeutic Touch, Reiki, lymphedema massage, cranial sacral); Traditional Chinese Medicine, known as TCM, (acupuncture, Chinese herbs, chi gong); Aryuvedic medicine; naturopathic medicine; homeopathic medicine; and nutrition and diet (supplements, macrobiotic and other special diets, fasting).

Although you may not get support from your medical doctor for use of complementary types of medicine, remember it is your right to choose treatments that seem appropriate for you. You have the right to get as many opinions and as much information as you need to feel you are on the right course. And sometimes, this may mean more than one additional opinion.

It is also okay if you feel that you do not need another opinion. Some situations seem pretty straightforward both in terms of diagnoses and treatments. And, some individuals really want to just rely on their confidence in a particular provider.

Finding "Experts"

If you want another opinion, consider getting one from someone who is really knowledgeable about what is wrong with you. For many illnesses, there may be one or more centers in the country that specialize in research and treatment of your particular diagnosis. You should consider a consultation with someone at one of these centers if you or your health care provider has questions. Insurance will generally provide reimbursement for at least one consultation.

I have been repeatedly surprised by how accessible the "big names" are. My experience over the past five years is that almost all of these experts were willing to provide phone consultation to my husband, myself, and/or our local doctor even if we did not see them face-to-face. You don't have to be intimidated by the reputation of the expert nor the geographic distance.

Using the Internet

The Internet has become a wonderful resource. If you do not know how to use it for research, now might be a good time to learn or to find someone who can use it on your behalf.

The Internet can be a good place to get basic information about your illness, including who typically gets it, what causes it, what the treatment options are, and what the prognosis may be. In addition, you can find information about current clinical trials and relevant news stories. A good starting place is Medline at *http://medline.cos.com/* or Medscape at *http://www.medscape.com.*

Keeping Track of Your Own Medical Information

If you are the kind of person who wants to be actively engaged in medical decision-making, then it really helps to have relevant information about yourself and your treatment. If you ask, your doctor or hospital can routinely provide you with copies of blood tests, lab reports, pathology reports, and consultation records. If you get information that you don't understand because it is too "medical," ask for help in clarifying its meaning. If some blood count or tumor marker has changed and your doctor doesn't mention it, ask about it. If you have slides from a biopsy that need to be delivered somewhere for a second opinion, carry them there yourself if you can. If that is not possible, then make sure that the sending organization has a secure way to assure their arrival in a timely way. Believe it or not, these are sometimes sent by regular mail and can and do get lost.

You might think all this record keeping is not needed, but it can make a difference. I have a friend whose report on a routine mammogram suggested a biopsy, but somehow, no one mentioned it to her, and she learned of it months later when living with advanced breast cancer. My husband's bone marrow biopsy slides were lost in the mail and caused a critical delay in his treatment and necessitated another biopsy (a painful procedure). Remember, information gives you, and those who are treating you, power.

CHOOSING TREATMENT

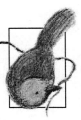

For many of us with life-threatening illness, making treatment choices is the single hardest part of what we have to face. The points below present just a very brief overview of a few key elements. One of the more helpful resources available is Michael Lerner's *Choices in Healing*, mentioned above.

Identifying What Is "Right" for You

Often, the choice of treatment seems obvious. This may be because there is standard treatment that is known to work. Or, it may be because you just knew from the start what you wanted to do.

In many cases, there is not a single "right" course of treatment. There are a series of approximately equal options, each with its own plusses and minuses. Or perhaps, there is no good option. Or, your doctor is recommending palliative[3] care only. Or, your doctor might be proposing something that doesn't seem right to you. Sometimes you may not know why the proposed treatment doesn't feel right; at other times, you may know precisely why it doesn't feel right.

When the choice is not obvious, it helps to try to clarify some issues that reflect who you are. Do the treatment choices have implications for what matters to you most? Will you have to be away from your family or have a prolonged stay in the

---

3. Palliative care is designed to maximize the patient's comfort. It does not treat the underlying illness or disease but rather the symptoms that interfere with a patient's comfort and quality of life.

hospital? Is there a mortality risk related to the treatment? If so, how do you feel about trading that risk off against what you have now? Is there a significant chance of compromised quality of life after treatment? How important is that to you?

Selecting a Provider or Providers

The provider you choose should match what you think you need, whether it is a medical doctor or a complementary or alternative medicine practitioner. Obviously the individual should be appropriately qualified to treat you and be capable of providing the treatment. But beyond that, there is a lot that can really make a difference in your overall health care experience.

For you, this may include a health care provider's willingness to be straightforward and direct with information. For others, it might be having the person with the best reputation, the "expert." For many, empathy and bedside manner are critical. Accessibility is probably central to most of us. What happens in an emergency? Who provides back up coverage? Can you reach your provider during non-office hours?

If you live in a rural location where a choice of specialists is limited or non-existent, consider asking your primary care doctor to discuss your treatment with a specialist in phone consultation. The specialist can be someone you see as needed, but not the one that provides your ongoing care management.

Selecting a Hospital

When choosing a hospital, there are a number of considerations. Is the hospital equipped to deal with your particular illness? For some treatments, for example, a bone marrow transplant, you would want to choose a facility that does a high volume of these procedures. For some treatments, an accredited community hospital would be fine.

In a tertiary[4] hospital or large medical center, you will have access to a broad range of specialists. This can be a tremendous advantage if there are complications. It is usually fairly easy to get a consultation with a doctor, often from a specialist who is used to dealing with your illness.

Staffing can vary tremendously between a community hospital and a tertiary facility. In a community hospital your own physician is most likely to follow your condition daily. Weekend and after-hours coverage will most likely be limited to a few people. In the tertiary facility, physicians are likely to change regularly and the doctor following you will probably be whoever is the "attending physician" for the unit. In addition, you may have medical students and residents who regularly see you.

You might also consider some of the less tangible things that may influence the choice of a hospital. This is particularly true if you are anticipating staying in the hospital for a long period of time. What are the visiting policies? Can someone stay in the room with you overnight? Are children allowed? Can you eat non-hospital food? Are there facilities for cooking or reheating food at the hospital? Are complementary medical practitioners allowed in the hospital? Are there supportive services available (yoga, patient support groups, meditation, etc.)?

If you know that your treatment will suppress your immune system,[5] ask the hospital about its policies and procedures. Practices regarding infection control vary

---

4. A tertiary hospital is one that is a major medical center, most often associated with a university or major research facility.

5. A suppressed immune system occurs because the immune capacity of your white blood cells is not working properly due to 1.) your illness (e.g. AIDS or blood and bone marrow disorders) or 2.) as a result of treatment designed to suppress the normal immune capacity or 3.) as a secondary effect of treatment designed to treat cancer.

widely among facilities. At one end of the spectrum, there are facilities that require everyone who enters a patient's room to be gloved and masked. That type of facility will often not let the patient leave the unit and limits the kind of food the patient receives to what is prepared by the hospital. At the other end, some facilities require only really conscientious hand washing and staying away from anyone who is sick. Which of these things feels right to you? Will they make a difference in how you experience your care? Do you have some preferences about this? Does your condition indicate what would be the most appropriate?

CHOOSING NOT TO HAVE TREATMENT

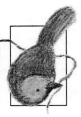

If you are facing a life-threatening illness, you may decide you do not want to have any treatment or you may want to have only symptom management (supportive or palliative care) or you may elect hospice care (end of life support).

How do you decide?

Try to start by sorting out some of your thoughts about what is "right" for you. Ask your provider if active treatment, for example, chemotherapy, is likely to extend your life? If so, what will be the cost in terms of your quality of life? How sick or tired might you expect to be? What complications can be caused by the treatment? This is particularly important if you are diagnosed with an illness that moves swiftly and for which remission or cure is not likely.

It has been my experience that physicians often prefer or recommend some active intervention in advanced cancer cases. It seems especially so if you are a younger patient. When you are diagnosed, you may be too upset to question the wisdom of these recommendations, but it is important to try. It may be the right thing for you to spend your last months of life primarily engaged as a patient undergoing treatment with all of what that entails (especially side effects) or it may be that you want to have as much of your normal life as you can.

If you decide not to pursue treatment, be prepared for the possible negative reactions of others. Some may well think that this means you have given up or are ready to die. And, of course, maybe some patients are. However, I suspect that most people who make this choice have simply decided that the quality of life in the remaining time is more important than the possible (but unknown) benefit of treatment.

GETTING SUPPORT

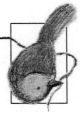

G etting support that works for you is essential to having a life as a patient with a life-threatening illness. As with making treatment choices, start with what will help you.

Identifying What Is "Right" for You

This is not necessarily easy. If you are a person who is private or likes to do things for yourself, you will have to figure out how to live through a period of time where you may not be able to go it alone. If you are a very social person, you may need to figure out how to limit or control your people contact, so that you are not overwhelmed or exhausted. Think about how to accomplish this before you start treatment. Ask a couple of people who know you well to talk it through with you.

You have never had to live in these circumstances, and you really cannot predict exactly what you will need. In general, however, it is probably safe to anticipate periods during your illness when you will need help physically and/or emotionally. So, even if you recoil at the idea, it may be helpful to try on the idea that support will be necessary.

Asking for Support

For many, if not most of us, asking for help is incredibly difficult. For some, it signifies they cannot do everything themselves, which may be something they pride themselves on. I have found it terribly difficult to come face to face with my own limitations. For some, it is the feeling they are imposing on others which is a difficult feeling to overcome.

So there are two really important things to keep in mind:

The first is that you probably will need help. If you try to do everything yourself, you may not have the needed energy for your body to heal. Or, you simply may not be physically able to care for yourself. Depending on your illness, you may need a lot, very little, or no help.

But the other thing is something that patients often don't consider. People who care about you want to and are gratified by helping. In the face of a life-threatening illness, many people feel helpless -- they want to help but do not know what to do. It is a gift you can offer to let others provide you with support. If you allow yourself to ask, you may well be surprised by the gratitude of those who are able – and want - to give.

There is an important caution here. Those you ask might not be able to provide what you need. Leave room for them to say "no." Individuals who feel manipulated into doing what you have asked or feel motivated by guilt will not give without some level of resentment. It is hard enough to ask, let alone be prepared to get a "no," but that is what you need to figure out how to do.

You may want to keep a running list of things that you could use help with. If you leave the list by the phone, it will be available when someone calls. Often when friends ask me what they can do to help, I can't think of anything. But if I keep a list, I tend to be more able to answer that question with a "Yes, how about . . .?"

Using the Support

There are many kinds of support that can be helpful. Below are just some of the things that might make a difference for you. Throughout this guide, you'll find lots of tasks that can be accomplished by a support person instead of the patient.

On the medical front, there is a wide range of support tasks that someone other than you could do:

Getting Information/Research. You might want help in understanding your illness, finding experts, complementary treatment providers or treatment facilities. At any point during the course of treatment, you might want to explore other treatment options. You may have a friend who is expert at using the Internet or a medical library. You may want to hire a person who works as a cancer counselor, guide or coach, someone who has in-depth knowledge about treatment options. Larger medical centers often have a medical resource specialist who can help.

Reviewing Medical Information. You may want someone to read and explain medical reports or help you think about treatment choices. There may be a friend or relative who has a medical or science background or who just feels more comfortable with medical language and who could explain the information. Medical terms can be incredibly confusing and another head can really help in understanding them.

Advocacy. You may want an advocate to provide support at a doctor's appointment or when the doctor sees you in the hospital. This person could help with issues of staffing at the hospital or with home-care providers. Sometimes, it is easier for the person who is not the patient to take a firm stand on something (with the patient's permission, of course).

Care Coordination. You may want someone to coordinate your care. This can be especially useful if you are unable to think clearly or to make your wishes known. Pain medication, chemotherapy, and surgery can all affect your ability to think clearly, so this is an item you might want to plan for, even if only on an occasional basis.

Transportation. You may want help with getting back and forth to the hospital or the doctor's office. This assistance may be particularly important if you are not feeling well. But, in addition, you may find the driving to these appointments particularly anxiety producing and some company can help.

If you are going to need to travel by air, either for consultations or treatment, ask your friends if they have enough frequent flier miles for a round-trip ticket and if so, if they would give them to you. And, depending on your illness, there may be some free transportation services. These services generally require that you be well enough to travel without medical assistance or elaborate medical equipment on the plane. You can locate these services via an advocacy organization for your specific illness (e.g., the American Cancer Society).

Assisting with Home Care. You may need help with your physical care. This can include organizing your daily medications, administering IV medications at home, helping with dressing changes, or assisting with medical devices you might be using.

There are also lots of non-medical things that others can help with.

People Stuff. Although it is a wonderful thing to have people who care about you, it can also be overwhelming. Managing the flow of people can be a place where you want/need help. There is nothing like being completely exhausted and having a steady stream of visitors or having a dozen phone messages you feel you need to answer when you are too tired for talking. It can be helpful to identify someone who can be the contact for your friends and family who want to know how you are doing. It can also be useful to have a person who can help you manage contact and visits with others. You'll probably find that people react well to the message that you need rest. Most people are perfectly willing to do something else (besides visit) that will help you.

Sometimes the people you are close to will feel anxious or afraid about what the implications of your illness are for their lives. You may not want to or be able to help them as you work through your own feelings. Sometimes, someone else close to you can do this on your behalf. On more than one occasion, when the medical news was not good, I felt overwhelmed at the prospect of telling friends and family members because I couldn't deal with their reactions and feelings. I could barely manage my own. This is a great time to have someone as your spokesperson.

Tasks of Daily Living. The many daily chores of just living may be too much for you to do at times. Getting support can make it possible for you to remain at home. Some of these tasks could include grocery shopping, cooking, house cleaning, laundry, running errands, transportation, making drug store trips, or mowing the lawn.

Things That Improve Quality of Life. There are other things your support folks can provide that really add to your quality of life. These can include giving you a massage, reading to you aloud, playing music or listening to music together, or meditating.

Help with Children. You may also want help with some of the things you normally do as a parent. This can include babysitting, taking kids out for some fun, helping them with homework, or transporting them to their after-school activities, medical appointments, and friends' houses.

Emotional Support. Getting the emotional support you need is critical. You will be feeling a lot. You may want someone to talk to, especially in the wee hours when you can't sleep. Or maybe, you need someone who can be with you when you cry or who can just hold you.

Finding Support

Sometimes it can be challenging to think about where to get the support you think you need. This may surprise you, but you have lots of options. Even if you think of yourself as a loner or you do not have any family available, there are places to get the support you need. Remember, many people will find the opportunity to help you to be something that they really want and enjoy.

Family and Friends. You will find that there will be some number of your friends and family who will immediately offer you support. One of the surprising things may be that those who offer will not necessarily be people you would expect to do so. There is something about the situation that may move some individuals to come forward and make generous and unexpected offerings.

Support Groups. You can probably find a support group in your area. It can be one for your specific illness or a general one offered by the local cancer organization or hospital. Ask your doctor, call your local hospital, or look in the newspaper calendar.

E-mail.[6] One of the great advantages of living in a cyberage is the ability to use e-mail to stay connected. E-mail offers some wonderful opportunities for support. You can feel and stay connected when you are physically far away or not up to seeing people face to face. You can read the mail when you feel like it and answer when and if you feel like it. I have been surprised that sometimes e-mail seems to provide an opening for some people I do not know that well to offer something really helpful -- maybe medical information or some relevant personal experience.

During both my husband's illness and my own, I have found it helpful to send out periodic updates on how we were doing to a large group of friends and family. These saved me having to repeat the same information, and perhaps more importantly, it really helped us to be connected to people who cared about us. I am repeatedly surprised at how much this has helped me to experience the web of support that exists but is so hard to see when you are isolated by illness. In addition, during Michael's illness, I often sent an almost daily update to my immediate circle of friends and family. Again, this helped me feel like I had support, and I did not have to retell the details of the day to a dozen people. You can do this via a group e-mail distribution. If you do set up a group distri-

---

6. If you do not own a computer, put the word out that you are looking for one to borrow. Often a friend or a service organization may have an old one that they can lend to you. Sometimes a local computer store may be willing to lend you one. If you can afford it, you may be able to rent one.

bution list, consider asking a computer literate friend to manage the names and addresses of the list as this can be tedious and consume a fair amount of time.

Online Support Services. Another computer-based way to get support is via list serves[7] or online chat groups. A great place to find a relevant resource if you have cancer is at *http://www.acor.org*.   For a non-cancer diagnosis, do a search that includes the name of your illness, a plus sign or the word AND, and the words "online support."

The great thing about list serves is that they can offer specific disease treatment and symptom management support. Participants are most often other patients and their families or caregivers although other individuals with useful information may also participate. Support can range from finding good treatment providers to learning about fast-breaking, relevant medical information, to emotional support, to finding financial resources or strategies for managing symptoms.

Patients with Your Diagnosis. I have found it very valuable to talk with individuals who have my specific diagnosis. You may find these individuals in a support group, by word of mouth in your community, or by asking your health care provider. If you have a rare condition, you may need to use the Internet to connect with individuals who share your diagnosis.

---

7. A "list serve" is essentially an e-mail that is distributed to a group of individuals who ask to go on a distribution list. When you subscribe, you generally have an option to get the messages for the day as individual postings or in digest form (one mailing daily that contains all the postings). I find the digest form easier to manage because it keeps the volume of incoming daily messages down. List serves have etiquette that is usually described when you subscribe.

Volunteers. Perhaps for you it may seem like there is no obvious person or persons to help with your support. Believe it or not, there are still resources. If you belong to a church, synagogue, or mosque, talk to your clergy. Even if you are not active, their resources will probably be available to you. Other places to check for support can be at your local hospital, your home health agency, or your American Cancer Society office. There are probably additional possibilities in your town that you can identify. Sometimes, when support people are not obvious, we overlook some possibilities. Do you have some work colleagues who might be available? How about people you know in your social or recreational life? If you feel reluctant to ask, maybe someone can ask for you.

A NOTE. One of the hardest things for some of us to accept is when individuals who we might have assumed would be available and helpful are simply not able. This can mean that people we counted on either do not show up or if they do, their presence is not helpful. This can be extremely painful, but it is not something the person with the illness can or needs to do anything about. Your health and healing need to be primary, and you need to let go of any guilt or anger you may feel when responding to those who cannot provide helpful support.

LIVING IN THE HOSPITAL

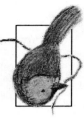

Nothing can strip you of your sense of autonomy and well being faster than being a hospital patient. All of a sudden it seems like you are your diagnosis. The focus of the nurses and doctors is on treatment, as it should be. Even though the care is not organized to maximize your quality of life, there is a great deal you can do to make the hospital stay work for you.

Managing the Medical Aspects of Your Stay

Although the hospital will not necessarily tell you this, you can be in charge of some aspects of the care they give you.

IV Pumps. While these pumps are great for feeding medications into your body, their alarms can quickly become a dreaded aspect of your hospital stay. The alarm sounds when medication is done and needs to be stopped or changed. However, the alarms have a tendency to go off at a lot of other times and often. The alarm has a way of repeatedly going off as soon as the pump is "fixed" and the nurse leaves the room. You can be waiting what seems like any incredibly long time for a nurse to come in and turn it off. This is especially troublesome when you are trying to sleep. Fortunately, the pump alarm has an "off" or "silence" switch. In my experience, most nurses are happy to have you silence the alarm as long as you call them so they can come back and check the pump and restart it. If the alarm problem continues, ask the nurse to find another pump. For some reason, these pumps are just temperamental.

Medication Schedules. It is not unusual when you are in the hospital to find your days and nights are filled with a steady flow of nurses arriving to give you medications. This can be especially irritating if you are trying to sleep. Most likely, you can change this. Ask your nurse to work with you to coordinate your medication schedule so that the number of times you get your meds is minimized, and you can get a good night sleep (or at least the best one possible).

IVs and Blood Draws. For many patients, there is nothing worse than getting "picked" with a needle either to draw blood or put in an IV. This can be especially true if you have difficult veins or yours have been used a lot for previous treatments. If getting picked is a problem, be sure and ask for the best nurse to put in the needle. Some nurses are really skilled at this.

Symptom Management. If you have a symptom that is bothering you, you have every right to expect and to get prompt symptom relief. If the medicine prescribed isn't working or the timing between doses is a problem, speak up. If a new symptom arises, mention it to your nurse who can then talk with your physician and make an appropriate plan. If you are not feeling well enough to do this, your advocate can be really helpful.

Understanding Your Medications. Either you or your support person should know what medications you are taking and should check that they are correct when they are being given to you. When changes in medications are ordered, an order can be inadvertently left off the chart or not reach the pharmacy in a timely manner.

Keeping Track of How You Are Doing. Remember you can have daily copies of all tests, reports, and notes kept on your condition, but you will probably have to ask for them!

Managing the Medical "Traffic." If you are in a teaching hospital or tertiary care facility, you may find yourself inundated with medical students, residents, and fellows. You may find yourself repeating your story multiple times. Or when a consultation with a specialist is ordered, the doctor who shows up may have a group of students in tow. If the "traffic" is too much, you can do something about it. You can ask your attending physician to arrange for a single person to examine you daily, and you can inform the consulting physician that only he/she is welcome in the room. This is absolutely your right.

Managing Providers. There are a number of circumstances where you may want to be assertive in managing your providers. Again, it is absolutely your right to do so. Particularly if you are in a general hospital, the staff may not be very familiar with the particulars of what your care requires, and you may need to remind or tell them about your specific situation. This is another place where your support person can effectively act for you.

If you require protection against infection, make sure that everyone follows the rules set up by your hospital. At a minimum, do not let anyone in your room who does not wash his or her hands first. You can put up a sign on your door that nicely makes the point that people need to obey the rules before seeing you.

If you have a port or catheter,[8] make sure your lab tech goes there first for

---

8. A port or catheter is a central line that is placed in your chest surgically. It allows for direct access to a major vein and eliminates the need for a lot of needle pricks to place IVs or draw blood.

blood. Also, make sure that it is cleaned according to hospital protocol by every nurse regardless of the time of day or the familiarity with the device. Nurses need special training to access your port or draw from your central line. In a community hospital, trained nurses are not automatically available.

If you have dietary restrictions, make sure the food on your tray meets your particular requirements. If not, ask a nurse to help you in getting a new tray that does.

Coordinating Care

When you are in the hospital, you usually have a number of different aspects to your care. Your providers may include nurses, residents, fellows, attending physicians, and consulting physicians. In addition, the pharmacy and dietary services will be involved. And you may have one or more complementary care providers who are not part of the hospital. These individuals may or may not actually see one another. They may work different shifts or in separate departments or in different organizations. It is in your best interest to make sure all the pieces of your care are coordinated to maximize the effectiveness of your treatment.

Rounds. Every day you can expect a visit from either your doctor or the doctor on the floor or unit. These visits or "rounds" are key times for you to ask questions, report new symptoms, and get information. This is a good time to have an advocate or support person with you. Many doctors are able and willing to plan their rounds at a time that makes it possible for your support person to attend. If rounds consist of more than a couple providers, this may not be realistic.

Coordination Among Providers. If you have multiple providers, particularly if you combine traditional and complementary practitioners, you will probably need to be assertive if you want your providers to work together on your behalf. This is important to making sure treatments are not at cross-purposes. It is reasonable to expect them to confer via phone or in person, but you may have to ask for that.

Coordination Between Shifts. Details can fall between the cracks when nurses change shifts. Feel free to ask the nurse on one shift to be sure and communicate with the nurse on the next shift. If you feel well enough, you can review information with nurses as shifts change, unless, of course, you are sleeping. If you have developed a strategy with the nursing staff for some symptom management that may not be mentioned on your chart, this can be especially important.

Nurse Assignments. It is helpful to have a relationship with the unit or head nurse as well as shift supervisors. If you have a nurse you don't like, ask for someone else. If you have a nurse who does something that really does not work for you, talk to that nurse directly or talk with the shift supervisor or unit nurse about the problem. If you have a nurse you really like, see if that person can be assigned to you regularly. If you are going to be in the hospital for an extended time, it helps to limit the number of nursing staff you are dealing with. That way, you can get a small team that knows you, and there is an increased likelihood that your nursing care will be better coordinated.

Creature Comforts

Just because you are in the hospital doesn't mean that you have to be uncomfortable. You can make life more pleasant for yourself.

Phones. There is nothing worse than a ringing phone just when you have finally gone to sleep. Here are two things you can do: you can unplug the phone when you go to sleep, or you can bring in your own phone that has a ringer you can switch on and off. If you use your own phone, consider one with an answering machine because it lets you know who has called but frees you from answering the phone if you do not feel up to talking. And you can even change the message so that the caller gets some information about how you are doing. Some hospitals require their buildings people approve any electrical device you use.

Clothes. Bring your own. There is no greater indignity than having to walk around in a "Johnny" with your backside hanging out. Bring pajamas, sweat pants and/or a robe that make you feel good and comfortable. Use slippers and avoid bare feet. Hospitals are incredible sources of infection and foot protection can help. Bring comfortable street clothes and put them on any time you are well enough to get out of bed for more than a few minutes. There is something empowering about wearing your own clothes. When I felt up to it, I found wearing a little jewelry and putting on makeup helped.

Food. If the hospital food tastes good to you, then this is not a problem. If it doesn't or you have special dietary needs, you have several options. First talk with the dietary staff and see what they can do to help you. At my local community hospital, they actually were willing to go to the local coop and buy organic food for me and prepare special meals. At tertiary facilities, this probably won't happen, but they may have some other way to meet your needs. Typically this might include foods that are not listed on published menus. Most hospitals have some facilities for patients or their family members to cook or warm food and refrigerators for storing food. Ask your support person if he/she can stock the fridge with foods that appeal to you or, possibly, actually cook for you. If you have friends that are looking for a way to be helpful, consider asking for some home cooked meals. However, if you are having trouble with digestion, appetite, or have dietary precautions, you need to be specific about what you can eat. At many hospitals you can have take out delivered in. This is great if you are craving a pizza or some Chinese food.

Room Décor. Make the room your own. Consider paintings or artwork that make it feel like home. If you have children, they can help you decorate. Put up photographs or get well cards. I actually had strings of beautiful origami cranes and some glittery stars that were draped around my room. I also managed to get a bird feeder put up outside my window. Too bad the birds never found it.

Other Comforts -- Music, Reading Materials, etc. If you like music, bring a tape or CD player with you. Something with headphones can be great if you are going to have surgery. You can listen to your favorite piece of music or a prayer or meditation, as you are wheeled off to the OR and during surgery. If you use a boom box, one with a remote makes it a lot easier for you to use if you cannot move around easily. If you like to watch TV, consider bringing a universal remote control with you since most hospitals have TV controls that only allow you to change channels by going up or down one channel at a time. And, if you are likely to experience diarrhea while you are there, think about bringing your own toilet paper!!! It can be a lot more comfortable. I found it was great to have my own pillow.

Visitors. While it is wonderful to have company when you are in the hospital, it can also be overwhelming. Consider posting a sign on your door. It might say: "Please check in at the nurses station before entering." (Make sure the nurses know how you want them to handle these requests.) Or "Thanks for stopping by, but I am not up to drop-in visitors today. If you want to see if you can arrange a visit, you can call- - - - -"

Creating Private/Quiet Time. Yes, this actually is possible. Talk with the head nurse about how you might be able to accomplish this. Often a sign on the door that says: "Please do not disturb, quiet time being observed until [insert a time]." Make sure it is scheduled so that it will not interfere with rounds or any other daily activity. I have been delighted to observe a group of doctors actually waiting outside a door until the appointed time. If you practice yoga or meditation, this may be the only way you can continue that practice while in the hospital. And, if you want to have an outside practitioner come in, for example to give you a massage, this is a great way to avoid interruptions.

Computers. If you are an e-mail user, take your computer with you to the hospital. It is a wonderful way to stay in touch with friends and family. You can read the mail and/or answer it when and if you feel like it. In addition, if you are on a list serve, you can keep up on information or post your own questions as you have them. If you are far away from your support people, this can be a great way to stay connected to them.

Exercise. If you feel up to it and are a person that wants to exercise, ask your nurse or doctor if there is exercise equipment available to patients. Some hospitals can provide aerobic or weight lifting equipment. If you have physical limitations as a result of your treatment, ask for a physical therapist to provide a consultation.

BEING AT HOME

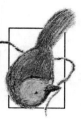

Managing the Medical Aspects

Managing your health when you are at home may be really easy or fairly complex. And it can vary over time. Like everything else about having a life-threatening illness, things don't usually remain the same.

Getting Medical Advice at Home. It can be frustrating trying to get the help you need with symptom management when you are home, particularly if you are far away from your provider or if it is after hours. If your provider is part of a large group practice, you may find the person you talk to on the phone is not someone you know. It may be another doctor who is covering for your doctor and who does not specialize in your type of illness. Or, it might be a resident. When you visit your doctor, ask if there is a way for you to call someone who knows you and/or knows your illness when your doctor cannot be reached. This may not always be possible, but it may be if you request it.

Symptom Management. If you have symptoms (for example, pain or nausea) that need active, regular, or periodic management, plan ahead. Make sure that you (and your support person if you have one) know what medications you can use, and how they can be combined. Write this down so that it is easy to recall if needed. Sometimes, when you feel really sick, you may have trouble remembering. Find out if there is a pharmacy that is open 24 hours a day. If transportation may be a problem for you, find out if there is a pharmacy that can deliver your medications if needed.

It can be hard to keep track from day to day, of what symptoms you experience. Sometimes keeping a daily log can be the best way to keep track and to review your situation with your health care provider.

After Hours Care. Make sure you know what number to call after regular office hours. As described above, talk to your doctor about how evening and weekend coverage is handled. Who takes the calls? Will the person have access to your records and/or be familiar with your medical situation? In large practices or those affiliated with medical facilities, you may be able to arrange to call or page a particular provider who knows you, but you probably have to ask.

Taking Medications. If your medication schedule is complicated, some organizing can help. You can make a daily or weekly checklist of what needs to be taken when and mark off the drugs after they are taken. It is amazing how confused you can get about what you have taken (or haven't) and when. Another approach is to make envelopes for the day or week. Each one should contain only the pills to be taken at a specific time on a particular day. The outside of the envelope should specify what drugs are in it, the dosage, and when they should be taken. When the medications are taken, the envelope can be thrown away. Another approach is to set a timer to remind you to take the meds. If you are having trouble keeping track of your medications, ask for help from a support person.

Medical Appointments. Go to your appointment prepared. Bring your questions, a way to record answers, and a log of symptoms and medication response. If you can, take your advocate with you. And, remember you can ask for a copy of any new medical reports.

Medical Care Coordination. Many professionals with different specialties may treat you when you are home. While you might expect they would communicate with you and with each other regularly so that your care is coordinated, it is probably in your best interest not to assume this. Make sure you tell your providers that your records and reports should go to your primary provider, the person coordinating your medical care. If you do not have a provider acting as the person in charge of your treatment, consider asking one of your providers to be this person. You want to be sure that all the aspects of your care are considered when a treatment or medication decision is being made.

Medical Care in Your Home. The amount of care you may need in your home can vary. The kind of care you may need can include changing dressings, maintaining ports or catheters, or cleaning wounds. Very often, these are things that you simply cannot do for yourself. Having some kind of help with medical care can mean the difference between being stuck in the hospital and going home. You may be eligible to have care from your local home health care provider. If not, see if there is someone in your support network who feels comfortable doing these things for you. Typically these are regularly scheduled tasks that your health care provider can train someone to do for you.

You may need help making your home ready for you as you undergo treatment or return from the hospital. You may need renovations so that your space is handicap accessible if you will be on crutches or using a walker or wheel chair. You may need furniture rearranged if you need a hospital bed brought in or other medical equipment. And, if you are immune suppressed, your health care provider may specify other special precautions.

If for whatever reason it is impossible for you to return to your home, talk with people in your church or community group about the possibility of some other living situation (assisted living, residential care home, or a room in someone's home).

Managing the Non-Medical Aspects

When you have a life-threatening illness and you are living at home, managing the non-medical aspects of living can be a challenging and, sometimes, overwhelming job.

Visitors. You may or may not want visitors when you are at home, and your preferences may vary based on how you are feeling at any particular moment. Just as when you are in the hospital, try to set up an easy way to manage the flow of visitors so it works for you. Let it be known (directly, via e-mail or phone messages to your network of friends) what your preferences are. Are drop-in visitors okay? Do you want people to call first? If you do not want drop-ins, consider putting a sign on your door that says something like "Thanks for coming by, but I am not up to visitors right now. If you want to find out how I am, call . . . . or to arrange a visit, please call . . . . " You might want to consider letting a support person coordinate this for you.

Remember that visiting with people takes energy. If your energy is low or you are recuperating, consider limiting the frequency, number, and length of any visits. If you do not have an advocate or partner with you, you might want to tell visitors in advance that it would be great to see them but only for some specified amount of time. Limiting the length of visits can be really difficult for patients who are very social, but you need to remember that your energy should go first toward your healing.

Food. Cooking can be overwhelming if not impossible because of your stamina or physical condition. Grocery shopping and food preparation are both fairly easy for others to do for you. And, remember, the people who care about you will feel better having something to do. If you have special dietary needs, or feel there are only a few things you might actually be able to eat, or have children with their own needs, let these preferences be known. I have even given my food helpers a recipe that my daughter really loves. You may not have the energy to organize instructions for food preparation and scheduling for meal delivery so see if someone in your support system can organize this for you. If you are not up to visiting with those people who are preparing the food, consider putting an ice chest outside your door where people can just drop off meals.

Church, synagogue, or mosque groups can often take on the responsibility for food assistance. And, check with your local social service agency or home health facility to see if you may be eligible for any local "Meals on Wheels" programs.

If you are going to have other people in your house putting groceries away or cooking, think about asking someone to label the shelves in your refrigerator and cabinets so the next person can easily locate food items. Make sure people wash their hands. Signs help.

Household Help. This can include all kinds of things that you may not be able to do yourself, such as loading and unloading the dishwasher, washing dishes, dusting and vacuuming, changing bed linens, mowing the lawn, snow shoveling, emptying the trash, etc. Again, try to start a list of what you need help with and keep it by your phone. When someone asks if there is something they can do, just go to that list. If you need help for extended periods of time, see if someone can take on a particular task for a period of time. Maybe someone can agree to see your lawn is mowed all summer or your sidewalk is shoveled for the winter.

Phones. In this day of answering machines and voice mail you have great tools for managing some of your social contact. If you are not up to talking on the phone, consider a message that says, "Thanks for calling. Please leave a message. I really appreciate hearing from you, but please forgive me if I am not able to return your call." You can also consider changing your messages frequently (or having someone do this for you) and providing an update on your condition. If you have more than one phone line, consider changing to the one that is less used (maybe one you have for a home business, a teenager, or an Internet connection) for talking with your close friends and family and then, turning off the ringer and using an answering machine on what had been your primary line. If you need to rest during the day or want to go to sleep early, turn off the ringers on any phones you are using.

DEALING WITH HEALTH INSURANCE

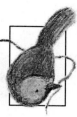

Even if you think that you have good insurance coverage, you will probably be surprised how much time and energy it may take to get provider invoices billed and paid correctly. You may want to consider getting someone else to manage this for you. If your energy is limited or if you just feel that you need to avoid the upset, find some assistance. There are people specifically paid to do this. To find a resource try your local Legal Aid office or office on aging. Some states also have advocates in the state departments of health or banking and insurance.

Working with Case Managers

Often the person who can help you the most is your insurance company case manager. Find out who that person is and get to know him/her. When you are frustrated with your insurance coverage, try NOT to take it out on this person. He/she is the person who can make things work for you so it is a good idea not to get into an antagonistic relationship. That said, if you feel like you are not satisfied with your case manager, remember you can always request someone else be assigned to work with you.

Getting Authorizations

For most life-threatening illnesses, you will need prior authorizations for some treatments. Make sure you find out how this process is supposed to occur. You may find your primary care doctor (not the specialist treating you for your current illness) has to make the treatment referral. Find out if your specialist can be authorized to act as your primary care provider for the duration of your illness. If not, see if there is someone in the specialist's office who can coordinate with your primary care doctor. On more than one occasion I found that a specialist never closed the loop with the primary care provider, but that there was an administrative person in the specialist's office who could take care of this. So, I learned that if I needed a referral, I needed to make sure this happens.

Understanding Your Bills

Probably nothing is as frustrating as trying to get your medical bills both billed and paid correctly. While it is often easiest to just pay your bills from providers when they arrive, it is probably going to cost you more than you owe. Before you pay a bill, make sure you understand why you owe it and how the particular amount was determined. If anything about the explanation does not make sense, question both the provider and your insurer. Some of the most common errors that occur include the following:

- The provider used the wrong code to describe the service.
- A referral was not made or was made to the wrong provider.
- The insurance company made a coding error.
- The insurance company overlooked an existing authorization.

Resolving Insurance Problems

If you get a bill or an explanation of benefits (known as an EOB) from your insurer that you do not understand, ask questions. Do not necessarily assume a bill or the amount paid by an insurer is correct. It may or may not be. Errors happen with surprising frequency. Make sure to hold onto any bills or EOBs if you have questions.

If you need to resolve insurance problems, create some simple system to keep track of your efforts to resolve things. When you make a phone inquiry, record the date, who you talked with, and what were the agreed to next steps. If you pursue information in writing, make sure to keep copies of all correspondence.

You have a right to understand your bills and verify that they are correct BEFORE you pay them. Keep asking questions until you get an answer that makes sense. If you think the person you are dealing with is incorrect, ask for an explanation in writing, and/or ask to speak with that person's supervisor. It is generally not advisable to pay a bill that you feel is incorrect, but be aware non-payment can lead to your bill being sent out to collections.

Filing a Complaint

If you cannot get a satisfactory resolution to your questions or problems, follow your insurance company's procedures for filing a grievance. Most companies will have a timeline set by state regulation within which they must respond. And, most also have an appeal process if you are not satisfied with the grievance decision

When you file a complaint, try to be succinct but include all of the relevant details. It is always a good idea to get someone else to review your letter before you send it. These are emotional issues, and sometimes we are not as clear or convincing as we might normally be.

Finding Assistance Beyond Your Insurance Company

In most states, you have another place to go with a formal complaint if you are not satisfied with how your insurance carrier has resolved your grievance. To find out what resources are available in your state, contact your state banking and insurance department or your local Legal Aid office. In some states, there are also advocates available to help you get your complaints resolved.

Unfortunately, sometimes the best way to get problems resolved is to bring pressure to bear. This can include using someone with political clout (a congressman or local legislator) or getting a local newspaper or radio to tell your story. Sometimes, it makes sense to retain an attorney to help you resolve these problems.

WHEN IS IT TIME TO STOP TREATMENT?

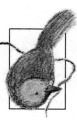

Deciding to end treatment is not something that is talked about often. But, when you have a life-threatening illness, it is definitely something you may want to consider. Although you may not be able to imagine that you would want to end treatment, if you allow yourself to try on the idea early, you are much less likely to make treatment decisions motivated by fear. And if the day comes when ending treatment might make sense to you, you may find it easier to make that decision. While it is not my intent to focus on end of life decisions, there are a few ideas that may be useful to think about as you live with your illness.

Why Stop Treatment?

There are a number of reasons to stop treatment. It may be that the treatment available is no longer working, and there are no reasonable alternatives. Or, the treatment is causing side effects that do not seem to be worth the perceived benefit of treatment. Or the treatment compromises your quality of life in a way that does not seem worth the potential advantage of continuing. Maybe you have to stay in the hospital and be away from your family to get treatment. Maybe you need to go to a clinic every day or have a home health nurse in your home for extended periods of time. Maybe the administration of the treatment interferes with the regular, daily activities you cherish. Maybe the treatment robs you of contact with what matters most in your life.

Lastly, you may simply be tired. Living with a life-threatening illness can be exhausting and sometimes it just becomes clear that the inevitability of death is not worth the price of warding it off by continued intervention.

What Is Right for You?

As with everything described above, the person with the illness is the ONLY one who knows what is right for him/her. This is completely an individual choice. Two people with exactly the same illness and prognosis, may choose completely different courses with one doing aggressive chemotherapy and the other going right to hospice care.   There is no single correct course of action.

If you have a life-threatening illness, the possibility of death will be your companion, no matter how you decide to proceed. All of the pressure on the patient to "think positively" can mean that thoughts about that possibility are pushed away. This takes a lot of energy and can add to your fear about what might happen. Hard as it may be, my own experience is that it helps to check in regularly and ask myself, "Does it still make sense for me to continue treatment?"

Planning for Your Death

Many of you reading this may not want to consider this section because it is too painful to contemplate. Again, my own experience is that the earlier you can think about this, the easier it is not to be afraid during the course of your illness. Somehow many of us have come to believe that allowing in the possibility of death means we are choosing it, or perhaps, giving up. If you can take a deep breath and allow yourself to think about death and even plan for it, the relief you may feel will likely surprise you.

Even if you cannot think about any other aspects of planning for your own death, make sure all appropriate legal documents are revised and in place (will, durable power of attorney[9] and living will[10] or advanced directive). If you have minor children and do not have a spouse or obvious guardian, identify someone who would be willing to care for your child and make sure that these plans are in a legally binding document. This makes sense for every adult, life-threatening illness of not.

If you can, think about what you want for end-of-life care. Do you want to be at home? Who would you want to be with you? Are there any particular things that might offer you comfort (hearing your favorite music or having a special comforter on your bed)? If you have an advanced directive, you will already have thought through what interventions you might want. If you do not have one, now is a good time to make one. Consider making sure your wishes are known to a spouse or friend who can see that they are honored. Again, this is something that every adult should have in place.

What kind of ritual do you want in remembrance of your life? Where should it be? Do you have a religious preference? Is there music or a reading(s) you want? Where do you want to be buried? Or would you like to be cremated? What would you want in an obituary? What about a headstone? It may be that you want to leave these decisions to those left behind, but perhaps you have preferences. Make sure these are known.

---

9. Durable power of attorney is a legal document that specifies an individual who can make medical decisions for you in the event that you are unable to do so yourself. It typically includes some guidance about your preferences.

10. A living will or advanced directive is a legal document that instructs your medical providers and those who care about you, what measures you do or do not want taken to keep you alive.

Talking with Friends and Family

If you decide to end treatment, you will need to tell the people close to you. Often your immediate family or friends will help in the thinking process that will lead to this decision. But, maybe not. Remember, it is YOUR life, and no one can make this decision but you. Only you will know what is right.

Do not be surprised if some of those close to you have strong negative feelings. A decision to end treatment can be extremely difficult for those who love you. It may be perceived as giving up (and it might or not be a giving up). Some individuals may even try to talk you out of it or ignore your decision by continuing to make treatment suggestions.

GOING FORWARD

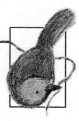

When you have a life-threatening illness, living is an incredible challenge, with high stakes and an intensity that you may fill ill equipped to handle. But it is possible to find your way and to maintain a sense of yourself.   The experiences you have will not be easy, and you will confront many obstacles but don't let that prevent you from having a life that works for you! By managing the practical aspects of treatment (both the medical and non-medical) in a manner that works for you, you can be *not just a patient* with a disease but your own person, uniquely you.

Acknowledgements

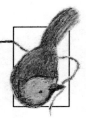

This book would not have been possible without a tremendous amount of advice and practical help. I could never list all of the people who have helped, but I want to offer my deepest appreciation to the following:

Sue Martell, head nurse at Fletcher Allen Health Care in Burlington, Vermont, who gave me the first hint that there was a different way to have a life in the hospital when my husband was sick;

Ellen David Friedman, organizer extradonaire and closest friend, who showed me how to let others help;

Rebecca Davison who encouraged and supported me to get this book written and published plus provided a "foster home" for my sweet dog, cooked for me, and was a caregiver;

Susan Sussman and Scudder Parker who gave my daughter a second home as needed during both Michael's and my illnesses and, with love, created security and safety for each of us.

All of my other "honeys" who helped in SO many ways. Dianne Maccario, as food queen and caregiver. Stuart Friedman as bill payer, surrogate on legal matters, medical adviser, and manager of frequent flier arrangements and much more. Erica Garfin as advocate and researcher, caregiver. Pat Fontaine who kept me in room decorations, clothes, scarves and accessories, and other accoutrements for the healthy spirit, who was a caregiver and as a cancer survivor, was invaluable in helping me with this book. The Seattle and Montpelier caregivers who included my folks, Harriet and Dick Fein, Larry Mires, Bruce Gratz, Leda Schubert, Bob Rosenfeld (who did NOT really change my clothes for me, despite his protestations to the contrary!), Andrea Serota, Rick Winston, Sandy Forquer. Jeannie Campbell, Coizie Bettinger, Gary Ireland and Anne Brand. I learned so much from each and every one of them.

All those who helped in reviewing and editing of this book: Janet D. Perloff, Ph.D., cancer survivor and Professor, School of Social Welfare and School of Public Health, University at Albany, State University of New York; Diana Peirce RN, Hospice Director Central Vermont Home Health & Hospice; Ginny Frye, author and Bereavement Counselor Central Vermont Home Health & Hospice; and Joyce Wolkimer, cancer survivor and writer.

David Ospina, MD, Elaine Owen RNP, Edie Fontana RN, and the staff at Mountainview Medical who have truly been my partners on the medical side of this journey.

Robert Brower who brought yoga into our home when Michael was sick. And all the other complementary and alternative providers, Arthur Makaris, Pamela Brady, Anita Rayburn, Smith Farm staff.

My spectacular daughter who has shown maturity, a sense of self, resilience and a tremendous capacity to grow through the challenges she has faced.

And Steve Worona who has filled my life with a love that has been a tremendous shelter on this challenging journey. And, who provided invaluable practical help --

managing my list serve, organizing medications, medical reports, etc., shopping, orienting caregivers, and caregiving himself.

And to the MANY, MANY others who have helped me along the way in Vermont, at Johns Hopkins, and at the Seattle Cancer Care Alliance in Seattle.

ISBN 155395860-8

9 781553 958604